We travel through journeys in life and
have control only on our reaction.

Battle with Grace
Cancer Doesn't
Define Me

Kelly McVicker

ISBN 979-8-89345-885-5 (paperback)
ISBN 979-8-89345-886-2 (digital)

Christian Faith Publishing
832 Park Avenue
Meadville, PA 16335
www.christianfaithpublishing.com

Printed in the United States of America

Contents

Day 1: Genetics..1

Day 2: Recognizing How Small...........................4

Day 3: Prepare for Battle 7

Day 4: Growing Concerns................................10

Day 5: Stripped Down 12

Day 6: The Move around Me............................14

Day 7: Together We Seek Prayer.......................16

Day 8: Give Up the Control.............................19

Day 9: Various Parts of the Battle....................21

Day 10: Reality Sets In..................................23

Day 11: Final Results 25

Day 12: Self-Image.......................................27

Day 13: Rooted..29

Day 14: Trust in the Lord...............................31

Day 15: If You Would've Been Here....................33

Day 16: Time of Rest.....................................35

Day 17: You Don't Know 37

Day 18: Generations of Richness.......................39

Day 19: Hiding in the Crowd 41

Day 20: Clothed in Strength 43

Day 21: Worship through Disappointments.........46

Day 22: Temporary Setbacks 48

Day 23: Scars 50

Day 24: Worship Team...52

Day 25: Anxiety versus Trust 55

Day 26: Unconditional Love 59

Day 27: Be Present 62

Day 28: He's Done Enough....................................65

Day 29: Family Disease 67

Day 30: Victory Is Ours 69

Day 1

Genetics

How many of us feel like our genetics have predetermined how things are going to end up for us? I am no different from others. I spent most of my adult years knowing I would likely one-day face cancer. My mother is a two-time survivor of breast cancer, and my father is a survivor of melanoma. Knowing your destination doesn't always result in preparing for the journey. On December 29, 2020, I went for my normal screening, the same as I had for several years. I had no worries and just strolled in and out, feeling like I was doing my routine check.

A week or so later, they called and said I needed to come back in for a diagnostic mammogram and ultrasound. Even at this point, I was not concerned because each time I went, they always wanted a deeper look. I said to myself, *They know my family genetics, and they are being thorough.* I went back, and they did the diagnostic mammogram first. The technician was moving me around and taking many images. Once she finished, they put me in a waiting room while the ultrasound technician prepared for me. I sat in the room alone, and the song "Battle Belongs" by Phil Wickham started playing through my mind. It was at that point I knew this was not the same.

The ultrasound technician came and got me. She went through some images and went to review them with the doctor. He came in and took his own images. They sent me back to get dressed and put me back in the waiting room. The doctor said we needed to do biopsies on both breasts and that the nurse would come and set that up. I went back for the biopsies and immediately scheduled an appointment for the results.

The day of the results, they contacted me again and said they needed a little more time. I already knew from my experience in the waiting room that this was the time for me to enter the battle of my life. The Lord doesn't send us into battle alone. I could feel a sense of peace all around. I cannot explain it, but there was a calming that could only be from the Lord.

John 14:27 (NIV): "Peace I leave with you; my peace I give you. Not as the world gives do I give to you. Let not your hearts be troubled, neither let them be afraid."

Day 2

Recognizing How Small

As the battle started for me, I, for the first time in my life, recognized just how small I was and just how big God is. Let's rewind a few years. For many years, I spent believing that if I controlled certain things around me, then I could avoid hard times. That is so far from reality. I would stress myself out trying to keep a spotless house while working sixty-plus hours a week. My husband would say to me, "Why are you worrying about that? Our house isn't even that dirty." That was something I could be in control of.

For the first ten years of being with my husband, we had separate accounts, and I paid the bills. Again, striving to control things so if something didn't work out, I wouldn't have to feel like I owed him something. The problem is, why would I even be entertaining that our relationship wouldn't work?

There was no indication that troubles were on the horizon, but can it really be that something would go as planned in my life? My daughters were exceptional kids, but I always kept them close, not trusting them to be around most people. These things I was doing subconsciously were feeding a great deal of anxiety in my mind.

I spent much of my life thinking I was big enough to hold back the waves of the storm. Storms don't come because we deserve them. The hard times teach us just how small we are and how good God is. He is a big God and wants to lead and guide us. We get in our own way. All this time, as I was going through these different situations, I was detouring myself and sometimes my family. People would say things like, "You're so strong." No, I was so weak and didn't even know it. Strength comes from faith. In ourselves, we are small, but through Christ, we are overcomers, victorious, and strengthened.

In this battle of life or death, I had finally come to the end of the line for Kelly. I had to lay it all down at the foot of the cross and trust that God was going to fulfill his will for my life. In that waiting room, he said to me that the battle belongs to the Lord and I have no choice now but to believe him.

Second Chronicles 20:15–17 (NIV): "15 He said: 'Listen, King Jehoshaphat and all who live in Judah and Jerusalem! This is what the Lord says to you: "Do not be afraid or discouraged because of this vast army. For the battle is not yours, but God's. 16 Tomorrow march down against them. They will be climbing up by the Pass of Ziz, and you will find them at the end of the gorge in the Desert of Jeruel. 17 You will not have to fight this battle. Take up your positions; stand firm and see the deliverance the Lord will give you, Judah and Jerusalem. Do not be afraid or discouraged. Go out to face them tomorrow, and the Lord will be with you."'"

Day 3

Prepare for Battle

As each of us recognizes that we are about to head into a period of change, we have so many different things going on in our minds and our surroundings. Some people will naturally start right into prayer, asking for guidance, and others of us will again try to "take care" of things in our own strength. When I say "others of us," I mean me. Once the news of the diagnosis settled in, I went straight into caretaker mode. I had several different doctors' appointments with a surgeon and a plastic surgeon. There was an entire whirlwind of questions, decisions, and information coming my way. In the midst of all this, I was worried about my team at work.

I spent the next weeks writing instructions for all the tasks I would normally do and making sure everyone was lined up to cover everything that needed to be done. It was like I was on autopilot. I had a great group of coworkers who willingly jumped at the task before them and did their part to rise to the occasion. I look back now at how I spent those few weeks leading up to my surgery, and I cannot believe the little amount of time I spent seeking the Lord. This is likely to gauge how much I changed through the process. Some of this may be due to that tugging feeling that the battle belongs to the Lord. After all, He did speak to me and cover me with an unexplainable peace. This is my first big journey, and clearly, I am allowed to make some mistakes through it. The caretaker mode made me feel like I was still in control of something. Is this healthy? It did temporarily take my mind out of spiraling mode, so it did serve a purpose.

As we approached my surgery, my husband and I had a lot of things that we determined we needed to practice. A double mastectomy is a very rough surgery for the first couple of weeks. With this surgery, you have limited mobility of your arms for a few weeks until the healing process starts. We practiced things like him putting on my seatbelt and washing and fixing my hair. My husband quickly mastered the flat iron. Again, I find it embarrassing that in this time, that was what I found to be important. I did find through this that my husband was a man of integrity and endurance. There was nothing he wouldn't do to get me through these weeks and months ahead. I was soon to realize the reason God selected him for me.

> Romans 8:28: "And we know that for those who love God all things work together for good, for those who are called according to his purpose."

Day 4

Growing Concerns

Even though many in my family had dealt with cancer, I still had no idea what the next days and weeks would contain. There is this natural feeling to let those close to you know what is going on. The truth is there are so many things that have not yet been revealed. The testing and technology these days are far different than they were when we went through this with my mom. The initial diagnosis was a tumor, invasive lobular carcinoma. As the weeks went on, the surgeon ordered an MRI, and I went back to get those results and found there was another section of cancer on the same side at the top. My tumor was at the bottom. Still trusting in the Lord.

The surgeon sent my biopsy out for genetic testing. The testing showed the cancer was a slow-growing type, and I didn't have the BRCA gene. It sounded positive, and I was thanking the Lord for this good news. On the day of my surgery, I was very calm up to the point where I had to leave my husband and roll into the surgery doors. This all occurred during COVID times, so my husband was the only person allowed in the hospital with me, and he never left my side other than when I went to surgery.

After I came to, I was told that the cancer had spread into my lymph nodes under my arm and in my shoulder. I had a much more extensive surgery than previously expected, but again, God is in control. All these changing situations years prior would have put me in meltdown mode, but I just keep remembering that the Lord spoke to me that the battle belongs to the Lord.

Psalm 25:5–7: "5 Guide me in your truth and teach me, for you are God my Savior, and my hope is in you all day long. 6 Remember, Lord, your great mercy and love, for they are from of old. 7 Do not remember the sins of my youth and my rebellious ways; according to your love remember me, for you, Lord, are good."

Day 5

Stripped Down

Do you know how life-changing it is when a control freak must completely hand all keys over to someone else? I had no idea how these days would forever change my mind. For many years, I prided myself on being the person who "takes care of things" at work and at home. Is it possible that everything continues when I step out of the situation? Well, that is just what happened. A double mastectomy was the path I determined was right for me. My family had multiple cases of breast cancer prior to mine, and years prior, I had decided if I ever faced cancer, the double mastectomy would be the route I would go. In order to take this path, I had to put all my normal duties in the hands of others. It's not that I ever felt that others couldn't do what I do, but rather I liked being the one in control.

I very soon found the world keeps turning even if you step out of the way for a minute. Up to this point, I really didn't feel bad. No pain, no big symptoms. People hear cancer, and they automatically presume you are very sick, and honestly, I didn't feel that way. This started the stripping down of who I thought I was and where I thought I was going. From that time on, I would start my days differently and spend my time differently. I was never filled with fear of dying. It seemed odd because everyone around me was feeling that fear. I don't know how to explain it, but I felt a great deal of peace and wanted to spend my days listening to worship music and healing. Many people will never experience having so much time to just sit and focus on themselves. It truly is a blessing, and for me, it was much needed. Prior to this, I would be that person who expected the worst and hoped for the best. I don't even know that person anymore.

Isaiah 55:8: "'8 My thoughts are nothing like your thoughts,' says the Lord. 'And my ways are far beyond anything you could imagine.'"

Day 6

The Move around Me

It's important to share glimpses of faith and love that surround us. One of the biggest impacts made on me was the swarm of love from family, friends, coworkers, community, church (mine and other churches), and friends of my family members. If you are ever blessed with the experience of people pouring out their support for you, then you truly have witnessed the power of the Lord. You might be thinking to yourself, *Surely not all those people were believers*, and maybe you are right. But I know what they did, and I know it was goodness. Those moments changed me forever, and I now look for opportunities to reach out to people and show support. It matters, and it is something that only costs us our time and a few kind words.

I received multiple cards every week and many gift baskets from multiple individuals and groups. I have every card to this day. I never want to forget those moments when people supported me and my family. My parents spoke many times about how impressed they were with the outpouring. People matter. You matter. Every day we can impact others in a positive and uplifting way. Look for the opportunity, and take the time to act on it.

> John 15:12–13: "12 My command is this: Love each other as I have loved you. 13 Greater love has no one than this: to lay down one's life for one's friends."

Day 7

Together We Seek Prayer

Going through my journey during COVID added stress to my family, but where there are difficulties, blessings and perseverance also reside. I want to share with you the posts from my family on the day of my surgery.

First is the post from my oldest daughter, Ashley. She wrote, "Please keep my mom in your prayers today. She goes in for surgery today to remove the breast cancer. We have faith God will see her through this, but we pray for a successful surgery and quick recovery. We love you, Mom! 🤍🤍🤍"

The next post is from my youngest daughter, Whitley. Whitley wrote, "Please keep my mom in your thoughts and prayers today as she goes into surgery today to get a double mastectomy. She is the strongest person I know, and I know God will be looking over her and the surgeons today as they remove the cancer, but it's going to be a long journey. Me and Ashley Hollows are going to be in the parking lot, showing love and praying around the hospital, but we would appreciate all the prayers and positive thoughts you can send our way ♥."

The next post is from my sister, Jessie. Jessie wrote, "It's been a heavy day. I have the strongest sister on the planet. Kelly Hill McVicker is fierce. She is a fighter. I can't even begin to describe how much she means to me, and I feel like I'm likely not alone in that sentiment. Never forget to tell those in your life how much they are loved because you just never know what tomorrow may bring!"

The next posts are from my husband, Shannon, as he tried hard to keep everyone up to date on the events of the day. He wrote, "Just wanted to update anyone interested in Kelly's progress. They just took her back for surgery." Later he wrote, "Things are going well. Reconstruction surgery has also started. Looking good for our fighter!!"

The last post from Shannon that day, he wrote, "She's finally out of surgery and in the recovery room. Both surgeons said things went well. I should be able to see her in a little bit. Thank you to everyone for the support and prayers, we sure needed it."

Reading through these two years later is so emotional. If you know, you know. In our family, we band together in prayer when things get rough.

> Deuteronomy 4:29–31: "29 But if from there you seek the Lord your God, you will find him if you seek him with all your heart and with all your soul. 30 When you are in distress and all these things have happened to you, then in later days you will return to the Lord your God and obey him. 31 For the Lord your God is a merciful God; he will not abandon or destroy you or forget the covenant with your ancestors, which he confirmed to them by oath."

Day 8

Give Up the Control

There is a great sense of calm once you realize you are not in control. Most of the time, we spend our effort trying to force certain outcomes. Think about this for a moment. We go to work and either put in 110 percent or 70 percent. Either way, we are putting in the same amount of effort we are expecting in return. Have you ever watched a kid on a team push and push when all along others know he just doesn't have the talent needed to get him where he wants to go? We force ourselves into careers, sports, relationships, and social settings that do not align with our path.

Once I was forced to be idle for my healing period, I realized all the things in my life I had tried to force. It was that moment where I had that light bulb moment of me not being as much in control as I thought I was. From there, my mindset changed, and so did my stress. Whatever is to come, I am trusting in the Lord.

> Proverbs 3:5–6: "5 Trust in the Lord with all your heart and lean not on your own understanding; 6 in all your ways submit to him, and he will make your paths straight."

Day 9

Various Parts of the Battle

Any battle we go through has twists and turns along the way. Is the day of the diagnosis the worst part? Is the surgery the worst part? Are the decisions the worst part? Is the unknown the worst part? Is the chemotherapy the worst part? Is the radiation the worst part? Is watching your loved ones fall to pieces the worst part? It appears there are more questions than answers. Each person has a different opinion of what is good, what is okay, and what is not okay. Even today, I am not sure which was the worst part, but I can tell you which was the best.

The best part of the battle is the comfort in knowing the Lord is with you, and you do not have to sway back and forth with the current of the waves. There will be really good days when one feels as if they could touch the clouds. There will be other days when you can hardly lift your head off the pillow. On both types of days, the Lord is our strength and comfort. No matter what tomorrow holds, we can rest in Him without fear of the future.

> Matthew 6:33–34: "33 But seek first his kingdom and his righteousness, and all these things will be given to you as well. 34 Therefore do not worry about tomorrow, for tomorrow will worry about itself. Each day has enough trouble of its own."

Day 10

Reality Sets In

About a week after my surgery, I began to realize that breast cancer wasn't my only fight here. Through the years, like most people, I had endured many times of trouble (some self-induced and some not). Throughout these situations, many protective walls were built, and I found that the more control I have, the more I can control the amount of hurt. This is a lie we tell ourselves to protect our hearts and minds. One week in, I wrote:

Right now, I sit here with very little control over anything. Not going to lie, last night and this morning I shed some tears. A little was pain-related, but most was because I cannot take control of this situation. I don't need to think I am in control… God is and always has been the one in control. As we go through situations out of our control, we learn to lean on the one with all the answers. He never fails us. He is our strong tower.

> Proverbs 18:10: "10 The name of the Lord is a strong tower; The righteous run into it and is safe."

Day 11

Final Results

Eleven days after my surgery, the results of the pathology reports came in. Out of fifteen lymph nodes tested, three were positive. My tumor's final measurement was 5.4 cm, which was bigger than what was measured on MRI. The second lesion on my breast was smaller than the previously measured 1.1 cm. With all this, the next thing to be done was a CT scan of the lungs, pelvis, and abdomen to see if it spread to any organs. The results of that could change the current plan if anything is detected. If not, we would move forward with the current plan, which was outpatient surgery to put a port in and start chemo and radiation to follow.

Each test and pathology report has been just a little different. To know the cancer spread outside of the breast normally would have put me into a very anxious state. You know, friends, we don't always get the path we want, but we do always get God's perfect plan. Shannon and I neither one shed a tear because we have faith in God for what he is taking us and our family through. This was a calm I wasn't expecting, but as the word says we are in the palm of his hand, and we can be still and know he is God.

> First Peter 1:7 (NIV): "7 These have come so that the proven genuineness of your faith-of greater worth than gold, which perishes even though refined by fire-may result in praise, glory and honor when Jesus Christ is revealed."

Day 12

Self-Image

As I walk around today, I don't view things the same way as I did before and even during my journey. A few weeks after my surgery, I was immersed in a mental battle over self-image. Like most people, I have struggled with this for a good part of my life, focusing on my imperfections. I have come to grips with knowing that living is more important than any physical appearance, but that doesn't mean that I just brush this off. The surgery wasn't particularly upsetting to me because no one would ever know if they just walked up to me, but knowing that in a few short weeks my hair would be gone was very impactful for me. I had asked my friends and family to pray for mental strength for these things when they prayed for me. The real battle was the vulnerability of others seeing me in a weakened state. Prideful? Absolutely! I had to walk through this so I could witness firsthand God restoring all things lost. Beauty is intended to be inner. It seems silly now how much of a battle this portion of the journey was, not being able to put the mask on and look tough. Oh, how the Lord knows each day what we need. The years of playing tough are slowly slipping away, and love will take their place.

> First Peter 3:4–6: "Your beauty should not come from outward adornment, such as elaborate hairstyles and the wearing of gold jewelry or fine clothes. Rather, it should be that of your inner self, the unfading beauty of a gentle and quiet spirit, which is of great worth in God's sight."

Day 13

Rooted

As we navigate through our journey, we need to find hope to hold onto, and for me, it was through scripture about "I shall not be moved." This is an important topic. We must be patient many times in our lives as we are trying to get to higher ground. Reflecting on my own life, I didn't have the career I wanted right out of school. I had to put in many years and work in many roles before I saw the benefit. I am rather thankful for this path as I met many people along the way, and it has given me a stronger support system while I endured my journey.

Life bounces back and forth within our little groups. Shared journeys and shared prayers lead us to compassion and love for our circle. Even people you have never met are touched by your circumstances and pray for you. When we watch others go through transitions that are scary or painful, we feel for them, but we are also watching how they act and react.

Trees are a good illustration of strength. As the winds blow hard, many times we will look out at the trees to see if they are still standing. The roots we cannot see, but they are holding the tree steady no matter the force of the winds. Jesus is the root, and no matter the journey, we can trust not to be moved by temporary winds.

> Psalm 1:3 (KJV): "And he shall be like a tree planted by the rivers of water, that bringeth forth his fruit in his season; his leaf also shall not wither; and whatsoever he doeth shall prosper."

Day 14

Trust in the Lord

One of the hardest things is to trust when you don't know where your path is going to lead. On the day of my CT scan, I realized that normally I would be worrying and desperately praying for good results, but that's not where my focus was that morning. God clearly said to me that the battle belongs to Him, and I am standing on this promise. If you know me very well, you know I have struggled with trust issues, but for once, I felt in my spirit that God was holding me in the palm of His hand. He didn't say you will breeze through, and He didn't say it would be a straight road, but He did say it is His battle.

It is such a relief to recognize that you don't have to fix every single thing that comes your way. Many of us want to be the fixer. It gives us purpose and power. It also wears us down and leaves us exhausted.

You know when you are little, and your parents are talking with you about something you are fretting over? You remember the relief when they say, "Don't worry. I will take care of that"? That's the kind of relief we feel with Jesus. Thank you, Lord, for going ahead of me and making a way when I don't see the way.

> Isaiah 43:15–16 (NIV): "'I am the LORD, your Holy One, The Creator of Israel, your King.' Thus says the LORD, Who makes a way through the sea and a path through the mighty waters."

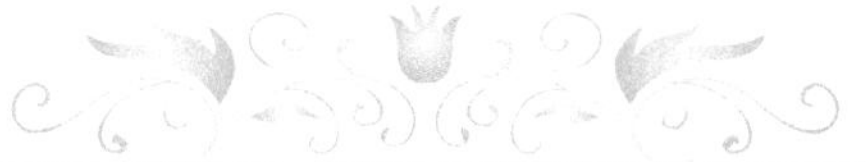

Day 15

If You Would've Been Here

Do you ever worry about not having enough to do? Being off work for long periods of time? Idle time was a real concern of mine due to my always throwing myself into work to escape what was going on in my head. A month after my surgery, I filled a lot of time relearning how to do many things in a slightly different way, and it kept my mind busy. I gained a whole new appreciation for people who have physical limitations. Most of us take for granted our unlimited mobility and youthful strength.

A few days ago, I was listening to an Easter sermon and heard a snippet about Lazarus, and even though I had heard the story many times before, this time I focused on Martha saying to Jesus, "If you would have been here, you could have healed him." Why is this significant? Jesus didn't have to be in the room and see what was occurring for His power to move. Many times we pray for what we know Jesus has done for someone else and not what He can do. We try to guide Him to a solution instead of trusting in His will for our lives. We pray for the situations that are a quick fix. Just like my physical limitations, I have been dealing with prayer limitations and not asking and believing for complete healing. Let that sink in.

> John 15:7–8 (NIV): "If you remain in me and my words remain in you, ask whatever you wish, and it will be done for you. This is to my Father's glory, that you bear much fruit, showing yourselves to be my disciples."

Day 16

Time of Rest

Have you ever been through a time when there was so much commotion? It could be health or grief or other journeys. There are so many things coming your way, and time just moves quickly through, but there will be a time when you are faced with your first time being by yourself. No one there but you and God.

My first day alone was spent listening to worship music. Little did I know this would start a new daily kickoff. The peace that comes with starting each day with the Lord is just what the doctor ordered. This often led to a powerful prayer for strength in my body, mind, and spirit. Little messages would come in from my team at work, which warmed my heart. Several occasions of comforting care packages connected so deeply within me to make me feel thought of and loved. This, too, would change the way I would react when seeing someone facing a hard time. One little glimmer of love will fill the heart and bring a smile. On my first day alone, I opened my devotional from the care package my church had given, and God reassured me to rest (scripture below). After all, this is His battle. After a few busy days, it is good to rest.

> Mark 6:31 (NIV): "31 Then, because so many people were coming and going that they did not even have a chance to eat, he said to them, 'Come with me by yourselves to a quiet place and get some rest.'"

Day 17

You Don't Know

As I sat thinking and preparing for the days approaching port placement and the start of chemotherapy, what came to my mind were footprints in the sand. This has always been one of my favorites because many times throughout my life, I know the outcomes were not always equal to my efforts, and as I get older, I have no doubt God carried me. Think about all the different emotions felt through many of those trials and how each one strengthened a different area. I had written a few days ago about self-image and losing my hair. There is something deeper here.

Right now, if I go down to the store, I can walk through there without a single person knowing I have cancer or that I just had a double mastectomy. My scars are hidden, and quite honestly, my muscles are responding well to the physical therapy. Do you see what I am getting at? There is a song by Zacardi Cortez called "You Don't Know." If you haven't heard it, you should look it up. It says, "You don't know what I've been through." We really don't know the things people are struggling with and don't want to share. How you feel about a situation can be completely different from how others feel about the same situation.

Finally, as I was thinking through this, I thought, *Why of all things is this the thing that is trying to stir some anxiety?* Then it came to me that it was a test of faith toward anxiety that I was delivered from.

deliver (Webster's Dictionary)
verb
past tense: delivered; past participle: delivered.

1. bring and hand over (a letter, parcel, or ordered goods) to the proper recipient or address

    First John 4:4: "You, dear children, are from God and have overcome them, because the one who is in you is greater than the one who is in the world."

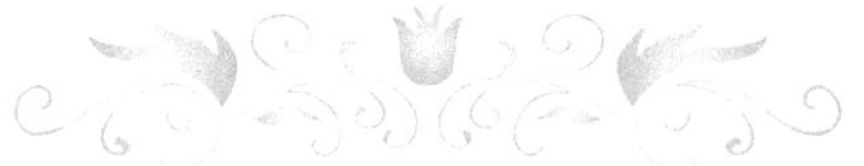

Day 18

Generations of Richness

When an opportunity comes around for a special gift, there are many items for order that have multiple generations sitting side by side. For my birthday, I received a picture from my daughter that started with my grandma and went through the generations down to my granddaughters. This triggered thoughts about the importance of grandmas and mothers.

My grandma was rich—not the CEO kind of rich. She was humble and truly a servant to her family, church, neighbors, and anyone else we would drag into her house. She had an unshakable love for Jesus, loved soap operas, and read *Reader's Digest* a lot. Most important, she loved deeply. She was a person who prayed for people instead of talking about them. She was never in competition with anyone and would serve others before herself. When I got pregnant at seventeen, there were two people I didn't want to tell—my dad and grandma—in fear of their disappointment. I remember like yesterday telling my grandma, and tears streamed down her face as she said, "You will be a good mommy." The love for family and love for the Lord has trickled down through the generations in the picture.

> Exodus 20:6 (NIV): "But I lavish unfailing love for a thousand generations on those who love me and obey my commands."

Day 19

Hiding in the Crowd

During my journey, I posted on Facebook, which was a recommendation from Martha, whom I go to church with. Putting out such personal and intimate thoughts was a bit scary at first, but honestly, when you are going through journeys, many people are curious about how you are doing—not just physically but also mentally and spiritually. As chemotherapy was quickly approaching, I knew soon my hair would be falling out. Hiding in the reader population was a girl I went to school with. We weren't particularly friends in school but knew who each other was. She reached out to me. She had really personal reasons for reaching out. Her family had just been through a battle with breast cancer, and it took the life of her sister.

I specifically thought of her when I started writing on social media because I knew the situation was still very raw for her, and I wanted to be very respectful of what was written. We had a couple of days of messaging back and forth about her sister and my writing. The one thing that she really did for me was to suggest that I take control of my hair loss—shave it off myself instead of daily having to go through the little-by-little loss and all the emotion. When the time came, my husband selflessly was the one to share the moment with. He shaved my head as we both had tears streaming. From that moment on, we moved forward from this part of the process and were more focused on staying out of the hospital through the chemo.

Relief came from a friend who was hiding in the crowd. She used her experience to help me. God puts different people in our paths for various reasons—sometimes for long periods and sometimes just for a season. My healing was contributing to her healing. What a big God! This taught me to be bold and reach out to people when God lays them on my heart. We have no idea what others are facing or dealing with, but we can trust that God knows the who and the how for a little bit of extra comfort.

> Psalm 91:11 (KJV): "For he shall give his angels charge over thee, to keep thee in all thy ways."

Day 20

Clothed in Strength

Life comes full circle, and you realize how instances years back resurface just when you need them. Eight years ago, I was struggling to deal with the passing of my friend Patti. She had pancreatic cancer that had metastasized from a melanoma. There were a few reasons that it was particularly difficult for me. First off, she was my confidant at work. I could tell her anything, and she would not judge. Also, she could always make you giggle and find positive vibes in every situation. The other thing I struggled with was that her boys were the same age as my girls, and I just could not fathom my girls having to face the world without me. This time was particularly hard for me, but I did learn a lot about death and grieving.

A good Christian friend of mine said to me at this time that everything that happens in your life prepares you for the next thing that is going to happen. No truer words have ever been spoken to me, and I often cherish that advice he gave me even to this day. During my journey, I thought a lot about Patti and how she handled her journey. She endured her battle with dignity and grace and kept on smiling. I totally get that now. At that time in my life, I had focused on a lot of the negative things around me (past and present). I really wanted to take that lesson from her and change my attitude. People talk about defining moments in their lives, and I always add this one to one of my defining moments. She had one of the most beautiful souls that I have ever encountered, and I am truly lucky to have known her.

Little did I know, a few years later, I would be facing the same battle and would need to hold tight to her example. She said to me that she had accomplished everything in life that she wanted, and she was at peace with passing. I now realize that what she was saying is we don't control our number of days, but we can be at peace with our lives. I strive each day to be true to myself and live in peace. Life is too short not to.

Proverbs 31:25–31 (NLT): "She is clothed with strength and dignity, and she laughs without fear of the future."

Day 21

Worship through Disappointments

The week leading up to my first chemotherapy, my mind was wandering, and I was focusing on something someone said, something else someone did, and something someone else didn't do. As I was worshiping, I started to really think about how I fell short and what God thought about me sometimes. Truth is, we all fall short. Then I opened Facebook, and my friend posted a meme that said God loves the drug addict as much as He loves the preacher. Some don't want to believe it is this way, but it is true. God shows us mercy and loves us no matter how big or small we fail. If He does it for us, then we should also do it for others. Pay it forward. I forgave some people that day who didn't even know they upset me. Don't be distracted by things that really don't matter. This only separates us from one another and, most importantly, separates us from God.

I was thinking back about something I read last week on how Jehoshaphat and his people went to battle (2 Chronicles 20:17) and God told them they need not fight in the battle and to take their position. The next verse says he bowed his face to the ground, and they worshiped. Their enemies in the battle got confused and wiped themselves out. In my next phase here, will you take your position with me, praising God for what He is going to do, and we will let God handle the rest?

Second Chronicles 20:17: "You will not need to fight in this battle. Position yourselves, stand still and see the salvation of the Lord, who is with you, O Judah and Jerusalem! 'Do not fear or be dismayed; tomorrow go out against them, for the Lord is with you.'"

Day 22

Temporary Setbacks

The surgery day came to get the port placed, and immediately the next day, I would embark on the chemotherapy. The evening before I started, I had a nice spaghetti dinner. Tomatoes are something you must give up during chemo. The journey pushes in the direction of doing a lot of things differently. Due to my surgery, I went several months without picking up my grandkids, took my first medical leave from work in over twenty years, and had to give up tomatoes too? Sometimes these little setbacks are like winding up a top. Once you take a break from something for a little bit, you really appreciate these things going forward.

With all the possible dangers of putting those chemicals through my body, I am concerned about giving up my favorite food for a few months. I giggle now thinking about it. The Lord knows the desires of our hearts, and He knows what we can and cannot endure. The whole journey is just a minor setback to refocusing my priorities and purpose in life. Wind me up, wind me up, wind me up. I came out of this journey stronger in faith and living life on purpose. Every day is a gift, and the temporary setbacks are a small price to pay for the return of many years of my life with a better vision.

Second Corinthians 4:16–18 (NIV): "16 Therefore we do not lose heart. Though outwardly we are wasting away, yet inwardly we are being renewed day by day. 17 For our light and momentary troubles are achieving for us an eternal glory that far outweighs them all. 18 So we fix our eyes not on what is seen, but on what is unseen, since what is seen is temporary, but what is unseen is eternal."

Day 23

Scars

During chemo, there was a lot of downtime to think, and I was looking at my new collection of scars until it really stirred me. I have been joking about my scars since my surgery—kind of my way of dealing with it—but today, I really started thinking about them. Just thinking about the definition of a *scar* in my words: a spot where an injury occurred and healed but not to its original state.

I started thinking about how my scars from the mastectomy wouldn't be seen much, but the scars from my port placement would. Scars should mean more to us—they represent what we have endured, and they should give us strength for the obstacles ahead of us. Are the scars we have sometimes for others? Do you think this is why some people's scars are visible and some are hidden?

Then I started thinking the scar doesn't have to be watched because it has already healed, but it is forever a reminder of what you have overcome, no matter how big or small. I have scars that were generated during times of weak faith and scars generated in times of deep faith. By appearance, they look similar, but the memories are a stark reminder that it is so much easier to get through holding the hand of Jesus. Nonetheless, I am glad to have reminders of healing and strength, so I always recognize that I am an overcomer.

Psalm 147:3–5: "3 He heals the brokenhearted And binds up their wounds. 4 He counts the number of stars; He calls them all by name. 5 Great is our Lord, and mighty in power; His understanding is infinite."

Day 24

Worship Team

Samuel isn't a biblical character we hear preached on much. Samuel was the judge who anointed Saul and then later anointed David in secrecy. Starting out, though, with the first chapter, I was guided to 1 Samuel 2: Hannah, who is Samuel's mother, starts the chapter praising in her prayers, which was the good word I wanted to hear, but I had to read on because my guidance was specifically about Samuel. Although I found the first part reassuring, I knew I could not stop there. Samuel, even as a child, had favor with the Lord, and that is what this chapter told of him. You may be more familiar with Samuel as the boy the Lord spoke to three times, and he thought the voice was Eli's. Eli had to tell Samuel that the voice was the Lord's. I thought back over my life and feel like I have always been shown favor too.

When I say favor, I am talking about God directing me out of situations that I didn't necessarily ask to be redirected. Quite honestly, I have made some very foolish choices, and they all worked for my good.

Fast forward to another day when I am directed to the book of Samuel, this time 1 Samuel 19. Samuel is much older now, and Saul is attempting to kill David, but the Lord touches Saul's heart, and he spares David's life. This is significant to me in the sense that no matter what things look like, one touch from the Lord and the situation will change. Later, Saul falls back into his old mindset and again sets out to kill David. Saul was wicked and persistent. Cancer is also wicked and persistent. Again, how did Samuel fit into this? The messengers that Saul sent out to capture David came upon Samuel and a group of people he was leading in worship. Their power of worship was so strong that it came over the messengers, even though they were not seeking God for the protection of David. I am going to have many different challenges in the coming days and months, but the things that come against me cannot withstand the group of worshippers on my side. When Samuel first heard from the Lord, he didn't recognize it, and these were dark spiritual times that were going to get darker. I think this is saying to me that things are going to get rougher for me, but listen for the Lord's voice and know that it's him when he speaks, and with just one group of worshippers around me, the situation can be overcome. Thank you to the group supporting me…I need you! I had a very rough day yesterday, but I am refreshed today in my spirit, and this will carry me through.

> First Samuel 3:11 (NIV): "11 And the LORD said to Samuel: 'See, I am about to do something in Israel that will make the ears of everyone who hears about it tingle.'"

Day 25

Anxiety versus Trust

Well, this morning, I was really starting to see the death of my hair roots. Little by little, each day this week, I had noticed eyebrows, head hair, nose hair coming out, and as I shaved this morning, the stubbles on my legs were lessened. What I felt like was a battle last month, I have embraced this month. This, to many of you, may seem so minor compared to the battle I am in, but you see, I don't have anxiety about the battle. God told me from day 1 that the battle was his, and I trust him. The side effects or short-term symptoms have tried to creep in and stir anxiety, but I keep closing those doors. You see, if I allowed them to stay, those anxieties will multiply, and before you know it, I could be back to the height of my anxiety journey. I remind myself frequently that I was delivered from anxiety, and I am standing on it. Trust versus anxiety. Let's look at the two words. First, *anxiety*, which means worry, tension. Other words: *apprehension, nervousness, restlessness, uncertainty, unease*. Next, *trust*, which is belief in something true, trustworthy. Other words: *confidence, expectation, hope, faith*.

I was thinking back on my life this morning on many situations and where I had put my trust even as far back as a child. We put trust in family, jobs, Christians, friends, money, education, etc. We have expectations (trust) that they are going to get us where we need to go. Each time one of these things fails us (which the Bible has always said they will), then our trust is chipped away, and anxiety takes its place. Ouch! Over the first forty years of my life, I took every mistrust event and put it on a stone to build up my wall. Well, I found when you get yourself closed into "the safe place," it doesn't feel that safe. I remember just a few years ago saying, "Everything is going in my favor. I wonder what is going to come crashing down." Anxiety. This was the height of my anxiety…the place I thought was the safest.

Last fall, I really started working through this control issue and really started praying for God's will over my life and my mind that he would let me know my purpose and use me in a mighty way. I was really battling with division in the family, in the churches, and all over our country. The land of the free really isn't at all a place where we can be ourselves. Families don't stick together like they did in our grandparents' era. Many people now don't even give a thought to church. Nothing is resolved by division except lost time. Several people have told my kids, "Your mom has worked so hard to get where she is, and it breaks my heart to see her have to go through this." Friends, for the first time in my life, I don't feel like this is punishment. I know the days ahead may roar like the ocean during a hurricane, but I know a God that calmed the sea with just a few words: "Quiet. Be still." When side effects try to attach to the anxiety blocks, I will be claiming, "Quiet. Be still."

> Mark 4:37–39: "37 A furious squall came up, and the waves broke over the boat, so that it was nearly swamped. 38 Jesus was in the stern, sleeping on a cushion. The disciples woke him and said to him, 'Teacher, don't you care if we drown?' 39 He got

up, rebuked the wind and said to the waves, 'Quiet! Be still!' Then the wind died down and it was completely calm."

Day 26

Unconditional Love

Looking back on the last several months, I am so thankful for God's grace. I am not going to lie; it hasn't been easy, but it has been relatively smooth, and I have had everything I needed. Why do these things happen? Many times, I believe it's an opportunity to gain closeness to God our flesh rebels against. The Lord is the same, regardless of how circumstances change all around. When we go through times of circumstances bigger than ourselves, we get a front seat to the faithfulness and goodness of the Lord. Some days, this is hard to grasp, but nonetheless, it is true. So many times, things happen at just the right time, and I wonder how many times we don't recognize it.

I had spent several days when my body was so weak. I woke up this morning feeling much better, but my body was sore from sitting/lying so much. I was really looking forward to the shower to loosen my muscles. I got in the shower and rubbed my head, and today is the day the stubbles come out. For forty-five minutes, I rubbed until the stubbles were minimal. I wouldn't have had the energy to do that in the past couple of days. I had worship music on and praised as I passed through this next step.

What kept coming to my mind the whole time was a situation a few days ago when I was so weak and lying in bed with tears dribbling down my face. My husband said, "You are so beautiful."

I thought to myself, *How he can feel like that when I am scarred up, the heaviest I have ever been, bald, and not able to do one thing for him?* Unconditional love is a blessing. We need more of this in our lives. We need to be able to see beyond people's shortcomings and sins and love them anyway. We are letting sin separate us, and not just the person sinning but the judgmental person on the other side is creating division too. Jesus loves us no matter what season we are in. He doesn't change.

First Peter 5:10 (NIV): "10 And the God of all grace, who called you to his eternal glory in Christ, after you have suffered a little while, will himself restore you and make you strong, firm and steadfast."

Day 27

Be Present

During the downtime, there is plenty of time to focus on values. I am like most people, getting wrapped up in work and/or work at home, and not spending time in the Word. I sometimes obsess over floors or laundry, which was a hard pill to swallow when I first had my surgery. I wish I had come across this scripture that a podcast led me to. Mary and Martha are Lazarus's sisters, but this scripture isn't about that. Jesus came to visit, and Martha did all the work while Mary sat at his feet. Martha complained to Jesus about her sister not helping, and Jesus told her she was worrying about things that don't matter and basically Mary had the right priorities. Wow!

I got three things out of this. First, we live busy lives—well, not me right now, but most of you do. We can make time, even if we must multitask or even if something doesn't get done. Stay in touch with God's Word—it's our shield and comfort. Second, Martha focusing on what Mary didn't do robbed her of enjoying her visit with the King of kings. This could have been me this morning as well. The washer is going, and so is the dishwasher, and I have the dog in here chasing the broom as I sweep, but none of that stopped me from hearing this word. Thank you, Lord, for meeting me today and giving me a good lesson on focus and priorities, encouraging me along the journey. Third, Martha focused on doing good works, preparing for the visit, and being hospitable but missed her time with Jesus. We can do many good things, and that is wonderful, but we can't leave out meeting with the Lord. The same goes for our families and friends. We must take advantage of the time we have in our relationships. We can feed the hungry and help others, but we must have that relationship with Jesus and our loved ones. Who will we call on when we are in need? We can go to church each week and show up for family events, but we need to be present and interact. I love good preaching as much as the next person, but the church is the people. I need these people on my side, and I want to be on their side. Same with my family and friends. I want you to be around when I am on the mountain and when I am in the valley. I want to be there for you in the same way. Those relationships will help us through.

> Luke 38–42 (NIV): "38 As Jesus and his disciples were on their way, he came to a village where a woman named Martha opened her home to him. 39 She had a sister called Mary, who sat at the Lord's feet listening to what he said. 40 But Martha was distracted by all the preparations that had to be made. She came to him and asked, 'Lord, don't you care that my sister has left me to do the work by myself? Tell her to help me!'
>
> 41 'Martha, Martha,' the Lord answered, 'you are worried and upset about many things, 42 but few things are needed—or indeed only one. Mary has chosen what is better, and it will not be taken away from her.'"

Day 28

He's Done Enough

I feel beyond blessed to have had only manageable issues during my time of treatments. There is a song by Beverly Crawford called "He's Done Enough." You should listen to it if you haven't heard it. Pretty much it says if he doesn't do anything else for me, he's done enough. How great is it to feel this way? It really put me in the mindset of a grateful heart. How many blessings can one person get? I think we all can have a joyful heart if we truly think of what blessings we have received, and not because we always deserve them, but just because Jesus is a good father and wants us to prosper.

It's easy for us to focus on something bad that happened to us and then spend the next years waiting for the next tragedy to hit, but this steals our joy and stability. Even in the storms, there lie many blessings.

Our lives are intended to be prosperous and happy. Our attitude and focus can change everything. Just as you want good for your children, he desires good for us!

Cancer is not a punishment. It is an opportunity to go deeper with God and open our eyes to the good days ahead of us. Praise the Lord for all he has done for me.

> First John 3:1: "See how great a love the Father has bestowed on us, that we would be called children of God; and such we are. For this reason the world does not know us, because it did not know Him."

Day 29

Family Disease

Cancer is a family disease, much like any big challenge you face. When my girls, Ashley and Whitley, initially reacted to the news of my cancer, I could so relate to their feelings because I also stood in their shoes with my mom. My kids have gone through a whole cycle of emotions and adjustments. They have their own busy lives to deal with and then cycle through the different stages as information and decisions come to us. They have been anxious, challenged, strong, searching, determined, faithful, and helpful along this journey, but life isn't normal for them.

My mom and dad have stepped in with comfort and strength for the girls and Sean (my son-in-law) throughout our journey, supporting Shannon and me with meals and visits and helping with errands, all while dealing with the emotional effects of watching their child battle. I have to say I am proud of all of them. Life really can switch lanes on you at any time. Each of us can say how we think we would handle it, but you truly don't know until you are at the bottom of that mountain looking up. I know one thing for sure: my hope is in Jesus. There is a reason they call him the Rock. Every day, every decision, and every obstacle, he was there for each of us. I am forever changed by his love and faithfulness.

Prior to my journey, I would worry about everything. Now the Lord has strengthened me to a place where I know my hope is in him and victory awaits.

> Psalm 62:6: "Truly he is my rock and my salvation; he is my fortress, I will not be shaken."

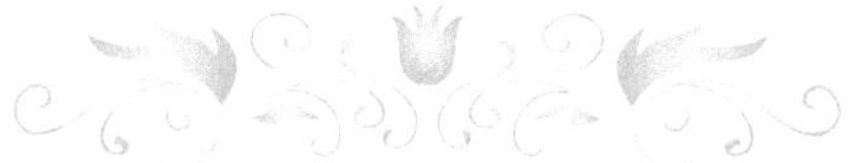

Day 30

Victory Is Ours

Just like that, the journey is over but not without substantial impacts. Life took a bit of a pause to teach me and many around me how fragile life can be and how victorious we are when we rely on Jesus for all our needs. From this day forward, I know victory is in Jesus, and my life will forever be changed. Each day, I will start the day in the Word and listen to worship music. There is a joy that only exists from His presence, and I don't want to spend a single day without it.

A lot of people fear cancer and the thought of how quickly things can change. With the Lord walking with you each day, there is nothing to fear. Take notice of how you spend your time and how you prioritize things in your life. Love those around you and forgive often. At any time, life can change direction, and as long as you are traveling with Jesus, everything will work out. He is my strength. He is my hope. Victory is mine. I didn't only learn how to survive; I also learned how to thrive. In the valley, praise Him, and on the mountain, praise Him. He is worthy of it all.

> First John 5:4: "For everyone born of God overcomes the world. This is the victory that has overcome the world, even our faith."

About the Author

Kelly McVicker cherishes her time with her husband, Shannon; daughters, Ashley and Whitley; son-in-law, Sean; and grandkids, Carly and Olivia. She also enjoys listening to music, crocheting, and quilting and loves the challenge of 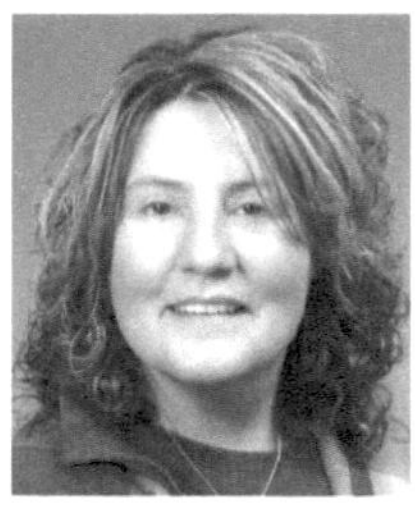 solving puzzles of any kind. She has worked in medical device manufacturing for nearly thirty years and enjoys serving her local community in a small town in Indiana.

Her love for writing sparked after sharing her journey through breast cancer on social media. She is passionate about sharing her source of strength, grace, and peace through inspirational writings.